Strength Training For Seniors Over 60

The Complete Step-By-Step Guide To Prevent Falls, Build Muscle, Enhance Stability, Improve Fitness And Balance (30-Day Workout Plan)

Karen Alexandra

TABLE OF CONTENTS

Core Workouts

- ○ Plank Variations
- ○ Seated Twists
- ○ Standing Side Crunches make it 10

Indoor Lower And Upper Body Strength Workouts

Outdoor Lower And Upper Body Strength Workouts

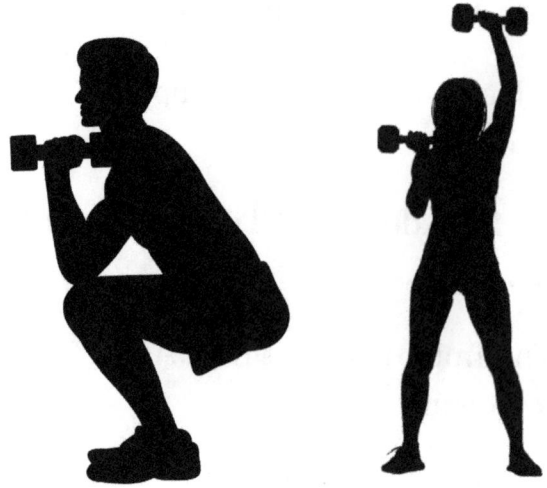

INTRODUCTION

Welcome to a world where power is more than simply physical; it is a mindset. We don't just lift weights here; we push ourselves to our full capacity, proving that age is just a number. This isn't about chasing youth or going back in time; it's about creating a legacy of vitality, one motivating workout at a time.

Imagine entering a setting where every movement is a powerful declaration of resilience. You're not just lifting dumbbells; you're breaking barriers and rewriting the rules of age with each repetition. This is not a grind; it is a celebration. Each press, curl, and squat represents determination and self-love, serving as a powerful reminder that your finest days are still to come.

Feel the excitement, laughter, and camaraderie of a community driven by a common purpose. Together, we turn problems into achievements, finding delight in every step of the way. It is not about perfection, but about growth. With each session, we mold more than just our bodies; we create a future in which strength, balance, and energy are our greatest allies.

Here, the gym transforms into a playground of possibility, with weights serving as transformation tools. Every rep is a spark of inspiration, igniting a life of confidence, energy, and limitless adventure. This is more than just strength training; it's a declaration that the best is still to come.

Join us as we reinvent what it means to age.With each lift, we demonstrate that life does not slow down,it grows stronger, more lively, and full of new opportunities. Let's thrive together, one exciting workout at a time.

WHY DOES STRENGTH TRAINING MATTER AFTER 60?

Aging is unavoidable, but how we age is something we can control. Strength training beyond 60 is more than just lifting weights; it's about improving your quality of life. Here's why it matters:

Managing Muscle Loss (Sarcopenia)
Sarcopenia is the term used to describe the natural reduction in muscle mass that occurs with age. Without intervention, this can lead to weakness, decreased movement, and a higher risk of falling. Strength training counteracts this process by conserving and even rebuilding muscle, allowing you to remain strong and active.

Improve Bone Health
Strength training not only increases muscular mass, but it also strengthens bones. Lifting weights promotes bone formation, lowering the incidence of osteoporosis and

fractures, and guaranteeing that your skeleton is as strong as your soul.

Improve Balance And Prevent Falls
Falls are the biggest cause of injury among elderly. Strength training minimizes the chance of falls by developing muscle strength, coordination, and stability, allowing you to take each step with confidence.

Improving Metabolism And Weight Management
Muscle is metabolically active tissue, meaning it consumes calories even while at rest. Strength exercise boosts your metabolism, aids in weight management, and lowers your risk of chronic illnesses such as diabetes.

Improving Joint Health And Reducing Pain
Strength exercise increases the muscles surrounding joints, improving support and relieving arthritis and other age-related

discomfort. It allows you to move with minimal discomfort.

Improving Mental Health And Cognitive Function

Exercise improves mood by generating endorphins, which reduce tension and anxiety. According to research, strength exercise enhances memory, focus, and overall cognitive health, allowing you to maintain your mind as sharp as your body.

Encourages Independence And Longevity

Strong muscles allow you to continue enjoying your favorite pastimes, such as gardening and playing with grandchildren. Strength training encourages independence, so you can live life on your terms for years to come.

Developing Confidence And Resilience

There is something tremendously powerful about gaining strength. Each session improves your confidence by reminding you that age does not determine your abilities—only your desire does.

Implementing A Positive Feedback Loop
Regular strength training boosts energy levels, sleep quality, and overall well-being, resulting in a positive feedback loop that benefits every part of your life.

A Lifetime Of Benefits Begins Now
It's never too late to start strength training. Every rep, session, and effort you put in is an investment in your long-term health, pleasure, and energy. Strength training not only adds years to your life, but it also adds life to those years.

BENEFITS TO YOUR BODY, MIND, AND INDEPENDENCE

Strength training beyond 60 is more than just a workout; it's a transformational experience that affects every aspect of your life. Strength training benefits physical health, mental resilience, and independence in the following ways:

For The Body

Boosts Muscle Strength And Mass
Aging naturally causes muscle loss, but strength training reverses this process by growing and retaining muscle. Stronger muscles indicate improved physical performance and a lower chance of injury.

Increases Bone Density
Lifting weights promotes bone growth, which lowers the risk of osteoporosis and fracture. Stronger bones help your body remain resilient and durable as you age.

Boosts Joint Health
Strengthening the muscles around your joints improves support, relieving pain from arthritis and other disorders while increasing mobility.

Increases Metabolism
Strength training promotes lean muscle mass, which burns more calories even when at rest. This promotes weight management and lowers the risk of metabolic diseases such as diabetes.

Boosts Heart Health
Regular resistance exercise lowers blood pressure, decreases cholesterol levels, and promotes general cardiovascular health, ensuring that your heart remains strong and healthy.

For Your Mind

Increases Cognitive Function
Strength training is not just good for your body; it also benefits your intellect. According to studies, it increases memory, focus, and overall cognitive function, which helps keep your mind fresh.

Lowers Stress And Anxiety
Endorphins, the body's natural mood boosters, are released during exercise. Strength training reduces tension, anxiety, and promotes a good attitude toward life.

Increases Sleep Quality
Regular physical exercise, especially strength training, improves sleep patterns, allowing you to fall asleep more quickly and wake up feeling refreshed.

Increases Self-Esteem
Achieving fitness objectives, no matter how minor, increases your sense of success and

confidence. You'll feel more confident and capable in all aspects of your life.

For Your Independence

Increases Mobility And Balance
Strength training lowers the chance of falls and accidents by strengthening important muscle groups and increasing coordination, allowing you to move easily.

Increases Daily Functionality
Strength training allows you to execute daily tasks with ease and comfort, whether you're climbing stairs, carrying groceries, or playing with your grandchildren.

Promotes Long-Term Independence
Strong muscles and bones enable you to live an active, self-sufficient lifestyle far into your later years, reducing your need for others.

Promotes Longevity And Quality Of Life

According to research, consistent strength training increases longevity and improves quality of life. It keeps you active, autonomous, and involved in the activities you enjoy.

Strength training is more than just exercise; it may lead to a healthier, happier, and more self-sufficient lifestyle. By committing to this practice, you are not only improving your physical and mental health, but also equipping yourself to face aging with strength, confidence, and vitality.

HOW TO USE THIS BOOK

This book is a thorough approach to strength training designed exclusively for elders over 60. It is intended to provide you with the knowledge, techniques, and motivation you require to reach your fitness objectives while maintaining safety and effectiveness. Here's how to make the best of it:

Start At Your Own Pace
This book caters to all fitness levels. Whether you are a novice or returning after a break, follow the step-by-step instructions and develop at your own pace.

Follow The Chapters In Sequence
Each chapter builds on the preceding one, from comprehending the benefits of strength training to mastering exercises and designing a specific workout plan. Skipping ahead may result in gaps in comprehension, so take it one step at time.

Use The Illustrated Guides

Each exercise is accompanied by vivid images and clear directions to ensure that you complete it correctly and securely. Refer to these visuals frequently as you gain confidence.

Use The 30-Day Workout Plan
The workout routine in this book is designed to help you gain strength, improve balance, and increase overall fitness. Use it as a guide and feel free to customize it to your own needs.

Remain Consistent
The key to success is consistent practice. Set aside time each week for your strength training regimen and watch your progress unfold.

Tips To Maximize
Your Results

Set Realistic Goals
Begin by determining your exercise goals, such as increasing strength, balance, or overall health. Clear goals can help you stay motivated and focused.

Track Your Progress
Keep a fitness notebook to track your workout progress, noting increases in strength, flexibility, and endurance. This will allow you to stay motivated and celebrate achievements.

Prioritize Proper Form
Maintain correct posture and alignment during exercises. This offers the greatest benefit while reducing the danger of damage.

Combine Strength And Cardio
Strength training can be combined with cardiovascular activities such as walking or

swimming to improve heart health and endurance.

Stay Hydrated And Nourished
Drink plenty of water before, during, and after exercise. To fuel your body, supplement your physical program with a well-balanced diet rich in protein, healthy fats, and critical nutrients.

Listen To Your Body
Pay attention to how your body reacts to each activity. Adjust the intensity as desired, and take breaks when necessary.

Be Positive And Enjoy The Process
Approach each workout with a sense of thankfulness and delight. Celebrate minor triumphs and remind yourself that you're improving your health and freedom.

CHAPTER 1

THE SCIENCE OF AGING AND MUSCLE LOSS

Aging causes various changes in the body, one of the most notable being the steady decrease of muscle mass, also known as sarcopenia. Muscle mass can diminish by 3-5% per decade beginning in your 30s and increasing after the age of 60.

Why is this happening? Several factors contribute to age-related muscle loss:

Hormonal Changes
A reduction in growth hormone and testosterone levels impairs the body's capacity to generate and retain muscle.

- **Reduced Physical Activity**
  As people age, they become less active, which contributes to muscle loss.
- **Changes In Protein Synthesis**

The body's ability to repair and regenerate muscle fibers declines throughout time.

But there's some good news: strength training directly combats sarcopenia. Consistently exercising in resistance exercises stimulates muscle fibers to get stronger, counteracting age-related decrease. This helps to maintain mobility, strength, and overall vigor.

The Relationship Between Strength, Balance, And Fall Prevention

Falls are one of the most common causes of injury and loss of independence among seniors. Strength training is critical in lowering this risk since it addresses the underlying causes of falls.

Increased Muscle Strength
Strong muscles give superior support for your joints and body, improving your ability to carry out daily tasks and regain equilibrium when destabilized.

Improved Balance And Coordination
Strength training exercises, particularly those that work the core and lower body, help to enhance balance and coordination. This lowers the chances of tripping or losing your footing.

Bone Health

Weight-bearing activities strengthen bones and lower the risk of fractures during a fall.

Joint Stability

Strengthening the muscles around your joints improves stability and alleviates discomfort, making movements more regulated and less prone to cause damage.

WHY THIS MATTERS TO SENIORS

Strength training is more than just looking fit; it is also about keeping functioning. Building and maintaining strength gives you the confidence to manage daily life more easily and independently. Strength training allows you to live your life to the fullest while reducing the hazards associated with aging, whether you're climbing stairs, carrying groceries, or enjoying your favorite pastimes.

CHAPTER 2

PLANNING FOR SUCCESS

It is critical to prepare oneself for success before beginning your strength training journey. Preparation ensures that your workouts are safe, effective, and pleasant, allowing you to reach your goals while reducing risk.

Essential Equipment For Home Workouts
Having the appropriate tools can greatly improve your exercising experience. Here's a list of necessary and optional equipment to consider.

Dumbbells
Start with a set of lightweight dumbbells weighing 1-10 pounds. Adjustable dumbbells are a fantastic choice since they allow you to gradually increase weight without requiring numerous pairs.

Resistance Bands
Versatile, inexpensive, and easy to store.
Choose a range of resistance settings to
accommodate different exercises and
progressions.

Stability Ball
A stability ball can be used for core
exercises, balance training, and as a
substitute for a bench in specific activities.

Exercise Mat
A cushioned mat offers support and comfort
for floor exercises, cushioning joints and
decreasing strain.

Chair Or Bench
A strong chair or workout bench is essential
for seated exercises, balance training, and
support during strength activities.

Step Platform
A step platform is ideal for lower-body
exercises that improve strength and balance.

Foam Roller(Optional)

Foam rollers promote post-workout recovery by reducing muscular tension and increasing flexibility.

Heart Rate Monitor Or Fitness Tracker(Optional)

These devices allow you to track your progress, your heart rate, and ensure you're exercising at a safe level.

How To Create A Safe And Effective Workout Environment

Choose The Right Location
Select an area with adequate space to move freely without colliding with furniture or walls. A 6x6-foot area is usually sufficient.
- Make sure the space is well-ventilated and illuminated for comfort and visibility.

Declutter The Area
Remove any obstructions, rugs, or things that may cause tripping or slipping. Keep the flooring clean and dry.

To ensure stability, use a non-slip mat or exercise flooring for your routines. Avoid slippery floors and uneven surfaces.

Organize Equipment
Store equipment neatly in a designated spot, like a shelf or storage bin, to avoid accidents and simplify setup.

Optional
Install a mirror to monitor form and alignment during exercises.

Maintain A Comfortable Temperature
Adjust the temperature to a point that is neither too hot nor too chilly. Staying comfortable allows you to focus on your workout.

Add Motivation (Optional)
To stay inspired, decorate your space with inspiring quotations, posters, or a playlist of your favorite peppy music.

Pro Tips For Success

Start Small
If you have limited space or funds, start with fundamental items like resistance bands and dumbbells.

Adapt As Needed
Your space and equipment can change as you progress. As your needs change, you can add or reorganize tools.

Test Your Setup
Before commencing a complete workout, perform a few moves to confirm that your equipment and environment are ready and safe.

CHAPTER 3

FUNDAMENTALS OF STRENGTH TRAINING

Strength training is not a one-size-fits-all solution. Each strategy provides distinct advantages, which you can combine based on your objectives, fitness level, and preferences.

Bodyweight Training
Exercises like squats, push-ups, and planks use your own body weight as resistance.

- Accessible from anywhere, no equipment required.
- Increases foundational strength and improves balance.
- Easily tailored to your skill level.

Chair-assisted squats, wall push-ups, and standing leg lifts.

What Is Resistance Band Training?
Exercises such as bicep curls, rows, and
lateral lifts are performed with elastic bands
with varied resistance.

- lightweight, portable, and
  inexpensive.
- Offers varying resistance, engaging
  muscles throughout their whole range
  of action.
- Reduces joint tension and increases
  strength.

Examples include seated rows, overhead
presses, and standing side steps.

Dumbbell training involves using portable
weights to enhance resistance to workouts
including curls, pushes, and lunges.

- Allows for progressive loading,
  increasing weight as you gain
  strength.
- Uses stabilizing muscles to improve
  balance and coordination.
- Provides adaptability in addressing
  certain muscle groups.

Examples are dumbbell chest presses, bent-over rows, and shoulder presses.

Importance Of Core Strength For Seniors

Your core is more than just your abs; it is a complicated network of muscles that includes your back, pelvis, and even your diaphragm. These muscles work together to support almost every movement your body makes.

Why Core Strength Is Important
- Improved Balance: A strong core stabilizes the body and reduces the chance of falling.
- Better Posture: Core strength allows you to maintain good alignment, reducing back pain and discomfort.
- Enhanced Mobility: Core muscles play an important role in everyday activities, such as bending down, tying your shoes, and getting up from a chair.
- Support For Other Activities: A strong core helps you complete

strength training activities safely and effectively.

Common Misconceptions About Core Training

Core training involves more than just crunches, including planks, bridges, and rotational exercises.

- Everyone may Benefit: Core training is appropriate for all fitness levels and may be tailored to your specific needs.

Core Exercises For Seniors

- Seated Core Twists: Sit in a chair with a light weight or ball and slowly twist from side to side.
- Pelvic Tilts: Lie on your back with your knees bent, then slowly tilt your pelvis upwards while activating your lower abs.
- Standing Side Bends: Hold a light dumbbell in one hand and lean sideways to engage your oblique muscles.

Bodyweight exercises, resistance bands, and dumbbells will help you build strength, improve your balance, and improve your general functionality.

CHAPTER 4

KEY STRENGTH-BUILDING EXERCISES

To increase strength effectively and safely, you must first prepare your body for the physical demands of your exercise routine.

Essential Warm-Up Routines

Warm-ups are not optional,they are necessary. They promote blood flow, boost joint mobility, and engage the muscles you'll be using. Warm-up exercises for seniors should be low-impact, simple to perform, and suited to their specific fitness levels. Each of the exercises given here has been carefully developed to deliver maximum benefit.

Effective Warm-Up Exercises For Seniors

Marching In Place

Stand tall, lift one knee at a time Swing your arms freely as you march.
Duration:2-3 minutes

Shoulder Rolls
Sit or stand comfortably.
Slowly roll your shoulders forward and backward 3 times.
Duration : 1–2 minutes

Arm Swings
Stand with your feet shoulder width apart.
Swing both arms forward and backward in a controlled manner.
Duration:1–2 minutes

Ankle Circles
Sit or stand while holding onto a solid surface.
Lift one foot and circle your ankle 2 times in each direction.
Switch feet.
Duration:(30 seconds per foot)

Seated Torso Twists

Sit on a chair, with your feet flat on the floor.
Place your hands on your hips or keep your arms at chest level.
Gently twist your torso to one side, then return to the middle and twist to the opposite side.
Duration :1-2 min

Toe Taps And Heel Raises

Sit or stand, tap your toes on the ground
Lift and press your heels back down.
Alternate between the toes and heels.
Duration:1-2 min

Dynamic Side Steps

Stand with both feet together.
Step to one side with your right foot Bring your left foot to meet it. Repeat on the other side, keeping a consistent tempo.
Duration:1-2 min

Neck Tilts And Turns

Gently tilt your head to one side, bringing your ear closer to your shoulder, then swap sides.
Slowly turn your head to gaze over one shoulder and then the other.
Duration:1-2 min

Seated Cat-Cow Stretch
Sit in a chair, with your hands on your knees.
Arch your back and gaze upward (cow stance)
Curve your spine and tuck your chin (cat pose).
Alternate slowly.
Duration:1–2 minutes

Leg Swings
Stand near a solid surface to maintain balance.
Swing one leg forth and backward in a smooth motion.
Switch to the opposite leg.
Duration:30 seconds per leg

How To Warm Up Effectively
- To ensure that your body is fully prepared, allow for a total warm-up duration of 5-10 minutes.

- Do each exercise at a comfortable, steady rate. The goal is to warm up rather than exhaust oneself.

- Take deep, steady breaths throughout the warm-up to increase oxygen flow to your muscles.

- Drink water before you begin your workout to stay hydrated.

Cool Down Exercises
For Seniors Over 60

Cooling down after a workout allows your body to return to a resting condition, minimizes muscle soreness, and increases flexibility.

Seated Forward Fold

Sit on a chair, feet flat on the ground. Hinge at your hips and extend your hands toward your feet while keeping your back straight. Hold the stretch gently.
Duration: 20 to 30 seconds

Standing Hamstring Stretch

Stand with one leg extended forward and heel resting on a low step or ground.
Hold your back straight and lean forward from your hips.
Duration: 20 Seconds per Leg

Neck Rolls

Slowly roll your head in a circular manner, clockwise for a few repetitions and then counterclockwise.

Keep your movements soft and controlled.

Duration: 10 seconds for each direction.

Chest Opener

Clasp your hands behind your back and gently lift them to open your chest.

Keep your shoulders relaxed.

Duration: 20 to 30 seconds

Ankle Circles

Lift one foot off the ground and rotate your ankle clockwise, then counterclockwise.

Duration: 10 seconds per direction, per ankle.

Overhead Side Stretch

Stand or sit tall

Extend one arm overhead and slowly bend to the opposite side, feeling the strain down your side.

Switch sides.

Duration: 15 seconds each side.

Seated Spinal Twist

Sit in a chair with feet flat on the floor.

Twist your upper body to one side, using the backrest as support.

Repeat on the opposite side.

Duration: 15 seconds each side.

Toe Touches

Stand with feet shoulder-width apart. Slowly bend forward, reaching for your toes without strain.

Do this lightly

Let your arms dangle.

Duration: 20 seconds.

Seated Shoulder Rolls

Sit comfortably and roll your shoulders forward for a few repetitions, then backwards.

Keep your movements smooth and controlled.

Duration: 10 seconds for each direction.

Hip Flexor Stretch

Begin in a mild lunge with one foot forward. Lower your back knee slightly to feel the stretch in your hip flexors. Switch sides. Duration: 20 seconds each side.

Wrist Circles
Extend your arms in front of you and form gentle circles with your wrists, first clockwise and then counterclockwise. Duration: 10 seconds for each direction.

Standing Calf Stretch
Place your hands against the wall. Step one leg back while maintaining it straight, then press the heel into the ground.
Bend your front knee slightly. Switch sides. Duration: 10 seconds each side.

Deep Breathing With Arm Raises
Inhale deeply and raise your arms overhead. Exhale while slowly lowering them to your sides.
Concentrate on calm, relaxed breathing. Duration:30 seconds.

CHAPTER 5

FALL PREVENTION AND BALANCE IMPROVEMENT EXERCISES

Single-Legged Stands
Stand up straight and position a sturdy chair or wall nearby for support.
Lift one foot off the ground while keeping your torso tall and straight. Hold the position for 3 seconds before switching legs.
Duration:3 seconds per leg (adjust as strength improves).

Heel-Toe Walks
Stand erect and position your right heel directly in front of your left toes.
As you walk, keep each stride as accurate as possible.
Duration: 1-2 Mins

Stability Ball Sit-To-Stand
Sit on a stability ball, feet flat on the floor, back straight.

Gently stand up, distributing your weight evenly.
Slowly sit back down while keeping control to avoid an abrupt plunge.
Duration:2-3 mins

Side Leg Raises
For support, stand near a wall or a strong chair.
Slowly raise one leg to the side while maintaining it straight, and hold it for a time before lowering it back down.
Duration:2-3 mins

March In Place
Stand with your feet approximately hip-width apart.
Lift one leg high in front of you, then lower it before raising the other. Swing your arms naturally with each step to work your upper body.
Duration: 1-2 Mins

The Clock Reach Exercise

Imagine you're standing in the center of a clock.
Reach out your arms to 12 o'clock, then clockwise to 3, 6, and 9 o'clock. Duration: 30 seconds To 1 Min

Flamingo Stands
Stand on one leg and stretch the opposing arm out in front of you to maintain balance.
Duration: 15-20 seconds per leg

Step-Ups
Find a solid step or low platform. Step up with one foot and bring your other foot up beside it. Step down one foot at a time.
Duration: 2 mins

Tandem Stance
Stand with one foot directly in front of the other, heel to toe.
To maintain balance, keep your body erect and engage your core muscles.
Use a solid chair or a wall for support if needed.
Duration: 30 Seconds per Leg

Ankle Sways

Stand with your feet shoulder width apart.
Slowly move your weight forward onto your toes, then back to your heels.
Sway side to side, moving your weight between your left and right feet.
Duration: 30-45 seconds

Toelifts

While standing, lift your toes while maintaining your heels on the ground.
Slowly lower your toes back down, keeping your action under control.
Duration:2-3 mins

Wall Push-Offs

Stand with your feet shoulder-width apart and about an arm's length away from the wall.
Place your palms against the wall at chest height.
Lean slightly forward and push against the wall to return to your starting position.
Duration:2-3mins

The Grapevine Walk
Step your right foot to the side
Cross your left foot over it
Step your right foot back out.
Repeat on the opposite side.
Duration:2 mins

Seated Leg Swings
Sit in a solid chair, feet flat on the floor.
Extend one leg and gently swing it forward
and backward while keeping the knee
straight.
Duration:2 Mins

Lifts For Opposite Arms And Legs
While standing, simultaneously extend your
right arm and left leg, keeping both straight.
Lower them back down and repeat with the
opposing arm and leg.
Duration:2 Mins

CHAPTER 6

FULL-BODY STRENGTH TRAINING EXERCISES FOR SENIORS

Upper Body Workout

Shoulder Presses
Sit or stand with your feet shoulder width apart.
Hold a dumbbell in each hand at shoulder height, palms facing front. Press both dumbbells aloft until your arms are completely extended,
then drop them with control.
2-3 repetitions
Duration:2 mins

Bicep Curls
Hold a dumbbell in each hand and stand with your feet shoulder-width apart and arms fully extended at your sides.

Slowly curl the weights toward your shoulders by bending your elbows while keeping your upper arms stationary.
Lower the weights back down with control.
2-,3 repetitions
Duration:2 mins

Tricep Extension
Sit or stand tall, holding a dumbbell in both hands.
Extend the weight over your head, then bend your elbows to slowly lower it behind your head.
Extend your arms back to their original position.
2-3 repetitions
Duration:2 mins

Lateral Raises
Hold a dumbbell in each hand at your sides.
With a tiny bend in your elbows, raise both arms to the sides until they are level with your shoulders, then slowly bring them back down.
2-3 repetitions

Duration:2 mins

Chest Press (with Dumbbells or Resistance Bands)

Lie down on your back on a mat or bench. Hold a dumbbell in each hand at chest level and press upward until your arms are completely extended before slowly lowering them back down.

2-3 repetitions

Duration:2 mins

Upright Rows

Stand with a dumbbell in each hand, positioned in front of your thighs. Pull the weights straight up to your chin, elbows higher than wrists. Lower the weights back down with control.

2-3 repetitions

Duration:2 mins

Arm Circles

Stand with your arms spread out to the sides, shoulder height.

Begin by drawing little circles in one direction for 15 seconds, then switching directions.
Repetitions: 15-30 seconds for each direction.
Duration: 2 mins

Front Raises
Holding a dumbbell in each hand, raise both arms in front of you until they are level with your shoulders, then descend them with control.
2-3 repetitions
Duration:2 mins

Reverse Flights
Bend gently at the waist while keeping your back straight.
Hold one dumbbell in each hand, palms facing each other.
Lift both arms out to the sides, keeping your elbows slightly bent, until they are level with your shoulders, then slowly return to the starting position.
2-3 repetitions

Duration:2 mins

Dumbbell Rows
Bend slightly at the waist and grasp a
dumbbell in each hand.
Pull both elbows straight back, compressing
the shoulder blades. Lower the dumbbells
back down with control.
2-3repetitions
Duration:2 mins

Lower Body Workouts

Squats And Variants
Stand with your feet shoulder width apart.
Lower your hips back and down as if sitting
in a chair, with your knees behind your toes.
Get back to standing.
Repeat 2-3 times.
Duration:2 mins

Lunges For Leg Strength
Step forward with one leg and drop your
body into a lunge position.
To return to the beginning posture, ensure
that your front knee is over your ankle and
push through the heel. Repeat for the
opposite leg.
2 repetitions per leg
Duration:2 mins

Calf Raises For Stability
Stand tall, feet shoulder-width apart. Slowly
raise your heels off the ground, landing on
the balls of your feet, and then descend back
down. Hold onto a solid surface for support.

Repeat 2-3 times.
Duration:2 mins

Glute Bridges

Lie on your back, legs bent, feet flat on the floor.
Lift your hips off the ground until your body is in a straight line from your shoulders to your knees, then descend back down.
Repeat 2-3times.
Duration:2 mins

Step-Ups

Locate a stable platform or step.
Step up with one leg, bringing the other to meet it, and then down one leg at a time.
Repeat with the opposing leg.
Repetitions:2 to 3 per leg
Duration: 2 mins

Chair Squats

Stand in front of a chair, feet shoulder-width apart.

Lower your hips back as if sitting in a chair, but do not actually sit down. Pause for a second before standing back up.
2-3 repetitions
Duration:2 mins

Leg Extensions

Sit on a chair, feet flat on the floor. Slowly raise one leg until it is straight, then bring it back down.
Repetitions:2 to 3 per leg
Duration:2 mins

Side Leg Lifts

Lie on your side, legs extended. Slowly lift your top leg to around 45 degrees before lowering it back down.
Repeat on the other side.
Repeat 2-3 times per side.
Duration:2 mins

Wall Sit

Lean against a wall, your feet shoulder width apart.

Lower your body into a squat position and hold for as long as possible.
Duration: 20-30 seconds

Core Workouts

Plank Variation
Begin in a forearm plank position. Keep your body in a straight line from head to heels. To vary the intensity, use side planks or plank knee taps.
Duration:15 to 30 seconds
Repeat 2-3 times.

Seated Twists
Sit erect in a chair, feet flat on the floor. Clasp your hands in front of you, twist your torso to the right, and return to the center. Repeat on the left side.
Repeat 2-3times per side.
Duration:2 mins

Standing Side Crunches
Stand shoulder-width apart, hands behind your head.
As you crunch sideways, bring your right knee closer to your right elbow before returning to the beginning position.
Alternate sides.

Repeat 2-3 times per side.
Duration:2 mins

Bicycle Crunches
Lie on your back, knees bent.
Bring your left knee up to your right elbow
while extending your right leg.
Switch sides to simulate a pedaling action.
Repeat 2-3times per side.
Duration:2 mins

Leg Raises
Lie on your back, legs straight. Slowly raise
both legs to the ceiling while keeping them
straight, then lower them back down without
contacting the floor.
2-3repetitions
Duration:2 mins

Deadbugs
Lie on your back, arms extended towards the
ceiling and knees bent 90 degrees. Slowly
lower your right arm and left leg to the floor
before returning to the starting position.
Alternate sides.

Repeat 2-3times per side.
Duration:2 mins

The Bird-Dog Exercise
Begin by kneeling on the tabletop. Extend
your right arm and left leg simultaneously
while maintaining them straight.
Return to your starting position and
exchange sides.
Repeat 2-3 times per side
Duration:2 mins

Russian Twists
Sit on the floor, knees bent, feet flat. Lean
back slightly and twist your torso from side
to side, your hands touching the floor on
either side.
Repeat 2-3 times per side.
Duration:2 mins

Reverse Crunches
Lie on your back, hands at your sides.
Bring your knees to your chest, then lift
your hips off the floor and towards the
ceiling.

2-3 repetitions
Duration:2 mins

Cardio Exercises

March In Place
Stand tall and march in place, keeping your knees raised to activate your core and legs.
Duration: 2-3 minutes

2 Step Touch
Step to the right and bring your left foot to meet it. Repeat on the opposite side.
Duration: 2-3 minutes

Walk In Place
Walk in place at a moderate pace to raise your heart rate while staying safe.
Duration: 3 minutes

Seated Marching
Sit in a firm chair and move your legs up and down one at a time.
Duration: 2 minutes

Side Stepping
Step to the right and bring your left foot to meet it. Repeat in the opposite direction.

Duration: 2 minutes ago

CHAPTER 7

INDOOR AND OUTDOOR EXERCISE ROUTINES FOR SENIORS

Indoor Lower And Upper Body Strength Workouts

Standing Dumbbell Press
Stand with feet shoulder-width apart, holding dumbbells at shoulder height.
Push the dumbbells overhead until your arms are straight
Lower back to starting position.
Repetitions:2–3 times
Duration:2 mins

Wall Push-ups
Stand at arm's length from a wall. Place your hands on the wall and lower your body towards the wall by bending your elbows, then push back to the starting position.

Repetitions:2–3
Duration:2 mins

Resistance Band Rows
Sit on the floor with legs extended, feet
against a door frame.
Hold the resistance band handles and pull
them toward you, squeezing your shoulder
blades together.
Repetitions:2–3 times
Duration:2 mins

Seated Leg Extensions
Sit on a sturdy chair, extend one leg out in
front of you, hold for 3 seconds, and lower it
back down.
Repetitions:2–3 per leg
Duration:2 mins

Dumbbell Side Raises
Stand with feet hip-width apart, holding a
dumbbell in each hand. Raise your arms out
to the sides to shoulder height, then lower
slowly.
Repetitions:2–3 times

Duration:2 mins

Chair Squats
Stand in front of a sturdy chair, feet
hip-width apart.
Lower yourself as if sitting down, but stop
just before your bottom touches the seat,
then rise back up.
Repetitions: 2–3
Duration:2 mins

Seated Marching
Sit on a sturdy chair and lift one knee
towards your chest, lower it, and alternate
with the other knee.
Duration: 2–3 minutes

Step-Ups With Dumbbells
Holding dumbbells at your sides, step one
foot onto a sturdy platform or step, bring the
other foot up, then step down and repeat.
Repetitions: 3 per leg
Duration:2 mins

Outdoor Lower And Upper Body Strength Workouts

Walking Lunges
Take a long step forward with one foot, bending both knees to about 90 degrees. Push off the back leg to step forward with the other leg.
Repetitions:2-3 per leg
Duration:2 mins

Step-Ups With Bench Or Stair
Find a sturdy bench or stair, step up with one foot, bring the other foot to meet it, and step down.
Repetitions:2-3 per leg
Duration:2 mins

Squat To Bench
Stand in front of a bench or chair outdoors, squat down to tap the seat with your glutes, then return to standing.
Repetitions:2–3 times
Duration:2 mins

Outdoor Resistance Band Deadlifts
Stand on a resistance band, holding both
ends of the band.
With feet shoulder-width apart, hinge
forward at the hips, keeping your back
straight, then return to standing.
Repetitions:2–3
Duration:2 mins

Wall Sit
Stand with your back against a wall and
slide down into a seated position, holding
the position for as long as possible.
Duration: 20–30 seconds
Duration:2 mins

Heel And Toe Walks
Walk forward for 20–30 feet on your heels,
then walk back on your toes.
Repetitions: 2–3 sets
Duration: 1–2 minutes each

Standing Calf Raises

Stand tall, holding onto a sturdy object for balance. Raise up onto your toes, then slowly lower back down.
Repetitions: 2–3
Duration:2 mins

Leg Swing
Stand next to a stable object for support. Swing one leg forward and backward, keeping your core engaged and focusing on your balance.
Repetitions:2–3 per leg
Duration:2 mins

Walking With Arm Swings
Walk briskly while swinging your arms to increase upper body movement and engage your shoulders.
Duration: 3–5 minutes

Outdoor Resistance Band Chest Press
Wrap a resistance band around a sturdy pole or tree, holding the handles. Step back, and press your hands forward in a chest press motion.

Repetitions: 2–3
Duration:2 mins

Stair Climbing
Find a set of stairs and climb up and down.
If necessary, take breaks between sets.
Repetitions: 2–3steps per Duration:2 mins

CHAPTER 8

CUSTOMISING YOUR WORKOUT PLAN

Tailoring your training routine to your fitness level is essential for progressing safely and effectively.

For beginners, start with simple movements like bodyweight squats, modified lunges, and chair exercises. Begin with 1-2 sets of 8-12 reps for each exercise.

- Prioritized Form:Learning good form is critical to avoiding injury. Make sure your motions are slow and controlled, and use mirrors or a workout partner to verify your form.
- Shorter sessions: Begin with 15-20 minutes of exercise, twice or three times a week. Gradually increase the duration and frequency as you get more comfortable.

- For Intermediate: Increase Intensity**
  Begin to use light weights, resistance
  bands, or dumbbells. Progress to
  exercises that work various muscular
  groups, such as squats with overhead
  presses.

- Increase Variety:Include a variety of
  strength, balance, and aerobic
  activities. To prevent tiredness,
  alternate upper and lower body
  workouts.

- Longer sessions:Aim for 30-45
  minutes three or four times a week.
  Increase your reps and sets as your
  strength grows.

Advanced

- Test Your Limits:You can now
  manage bigger weights and resistance
  bands. Include more complicated
  motions like single-leg squats, lunges
  with bicep curls, and compound
  workouts.

- Circuit Training:Increase the intensity with circuit workouts that include exercises such as step-ups, planks, and dumbbell presses, with little pause between sets.
- Full-body workouts:Aim for 45-60 minutes of exercise four to five times a week, combining strength, endurance, and flexibility exercises for overall fitness.

Listening To Your Body: When To Push Or Rest

Your body is the most trustworthy source of feedback throughout an exercise. Learning to listen to it helps you avoid overexertion and guarantees you're moving safely.

When To Push
- In Mild Discomfort:It is normal to experience a minor burn or muscle exhaustion when challenging your body. Pushing through a little discomfort helps you gain strength.
- Gradual Progression:** When exercises feel too easy, increase the resistance, reps, or length. However, make sure you're still using good form.

When To Rest
- Sharp Discomfort:If you feel sudden or sharp discomfort, stop immediately. This could imply strain or an injury.

Before you resume, consult with a healthcare professional.

- Fatigue or dizziness: If you feel lightheaded, dizzy, or particularly tired, take a break. Hydrate and relax to allow your body to heal before proceeding.
- Rested Days: Rest is essential for muscular recovery. Make sure you get 1-2 rest days per week to allow your muscles to recover and strengthen.

The Importance Of Recovery:Proper recovery through sleep, water, and nutrition promotes muscular growth and energy levels for future exercises.

Tips To Stay Motivated

Consistency is key for any workout routine, but staying motivated can be difficult. Here are some techniques to stay motivated, regardless of your fitness level:

- Set Realistic Goals:Set clear and quantifiable goals that are attainable. Having clear goals, whether they are to improve balance, increase walking distance, or lift a specific weight, helps you stay on track.

- Track your progress: Maintain a fitness journal or utilize a tracking app. Track your reps, sets, weights, and how you feel during and after each session. Seeing your progress over time can be quite motivating.

- Celebrate Achievements: Don't wait till a huge milestone to celebrate! Every minor achievement, such as raising your reps or feeling stronger in your regular tasks, is worthy of appreciation.

- Workout with a Partner: Look for a workout companion or join a fitness group. Having a friend to exercise with increases the fun and accountability, which can help you stay regular.

- Make It Fun:Mix up your routines to make them interesting. Try new activities, dance, go for a walk in nature, or enroll in a group class. The more pleasurable your habit, the more likely you will keep to it.

- Focus on How You Feel: Recognize the benefits of regular exercise, including improved sleep, mood, vitality, and independence in everyday activities. These rewards can be powerful motivators.

- Reward Yourself: Give yourself a treat after finishing a workout or meeting a fitness goal. Whether it's eating a healthy snack, taking a warm bath, or engaging in a hobby, rewards keep motivation high.

- Establish a Routine:Consistency is essential to success. Set a workout regimen and stick to it. Making exercise a part of your daily routine turns it into a habit rather than a hassle.

- Maintain a Positive Attitude: Do not get discouraged by setbacks. Every day represents a new opportunity to make improvements. Celebrate your perseverance and concentrate on the wonderful changes you are experiencing.

A 30-Day Strength Training Plan

Week 1

Establishing A Strong Foundation

Daily Routine
Warm-Up:5-10 minutes of easy cardio (e.g., walking in place or arm circles).
Strength training includes chair squats.
Perform two sets of 2-3reps of wall push-ups.
Perform 2 sets of 3-5 reps with seated leg raises.
Perform 2 sets of 3 reps per leg for

Standing Heel Raises
 2 sets of 2-3 reps
Bicep Curls with light dumbbells
Perform 2 sets of 2-3 reps.

Cool Down

5 minutes of mild stretching, focusing on the legs, back, and shoulders.

Weekly Focus
Practice appropriate form and become comfortable with the movements.
- Keep the intensity low to moderate, focusing on learning the routines.
- Rest days: As you get used to this regimen, set aside 1-2 days for rest.

WEEk 2

Improving Stability And Endurance

Now that you have a solid foundation, it's time to improve your stability and endurance. This week, you'll start introducing more variation to your workouts while strengthening your balance and endurance.

Daily Routine: Warm-Up: 5-10 minutes
Low-impact cardio (e.g., walking with knee lifts or side steps).
Strength training includes chair squats with heel raise.
Perform three sets of 2-3 reps of modified push-ups (on knees).
3 sets of 2-3 reps
Step-ups with a low step
Perform 3 sets of 3 reps per leg with

Standing Hip Abductions

Perform 3 sets of 2-3repetitions each leg
with dumbbell shoulder presses.
3 sets of 2-3 repetitions

Standing Leg Extensions
Perform 3 sets of 3 reps per leg. -

Cool-down
Stretch for 5 minutes, focusing on your hips,
hamstrings, and arms.

This week's focus is on improving balance
with challenging stability routines like
standing on one leg.

- Increase the duration of each exercise
  and aim for more reps.
- Rest days: Try to schedule 1-2 days of
  rest or active rehabilitation, such as
  mild walking or stretching.

Week 3

Increasing Core Strength And Flexibility

Daily Routine
Warm-Up: 5 minutes of easy cardio (e.g., marching in place or toe tapping).
Strength training includes standing oblique crunches. 3 sets of 3reps per side
Seated Marching (to activate core muscles)
Three sets of 3 Marches Bridge Exercise - Perform 3 sets of 2-3reps of standing or seated knee lifts for core activation.
Perform 3 sets of 2-3 reps per leg. Plank (on knees or against a wall). Hold for 10-15 seconds, 3 times.
Twist the torso while sitting or standing. Perform 3 sets of 3-5reps per side.

Cool-down
5 minutes of full-body stretching, with emphasis on the lower back, knees, and shoulders.

Focus For The Week

Practice core exercises to improve stability and balance.

- Increase flexibility by gradually stretching muscles after each strength training.
- Rest days: To ensure appropriate healing, try restorative activities such as yoga or stretching.

WEEk 4

Developing Balance
And Total Body Strength

Daily Routine:Warm-Up
Perform 5-10 minutes of low-impact cardio with side steps and arm swings.
Strength training includes chair squats with bicep curls.
Perform 3 sets of 2-3 reps with Lateral Leg Raises (to the side). 3 sets of 3 reps on each side.

Heel-To-Toe Walk
3 sets of 3 steps forward and back Step-Ups with Dumbbell Press. Three sets of 3 repetitions per leg.

Seated Row With Resistance Bands 3 sets of 2-3 reps for Standing Calf Raise.Perform 3 sets of 3 reps.

Cool-down

5-minutes of stretching, focusing on the back, hips, and legs.

This week's focus is on strength and balance exercises, such as heel-toe walking and weighted step-ups.

- Use movements that require coordination and core control to improve balance.
- Rest days: Schedule 1-2 full rest days or active recovery activities (such as walking, stretching, or swimming).

CHAPTER 9

NUTRITION FOR STRENGTH AND RECOVERY

Nutrition is more than just eating; it is about feeding your body so that it can work well and recuperate efficiently.

The Importance Of Protein In Muscle Building

Protein is the building block of muscle, and as we get older, it's even more crucial to eat enough to maintain and develop muscle mass. Consuming a proper amount of protein can assist seniors maintain muscle strength, heal tissues, and improve recovery time after workouts.

- Why Protein Matters: Protein promotes muscle repair and growth by repairing micro-tears in muscle fibers caused by strength training, leading to stronger and more resilient muscles.

- Protecting Muscle Mass:Muscle mass naturally reduces with aging. Consuming enough protein can halt the process and possibly assist create new muscle.
- Increasing Metabolism:Protein can assist maintain a healthy metabolism, which is essential for weight management and energy levels.

The recommended daily protein intake for seniors is 1.0 to 1.2 grams per kilogram of body weight. For example, a 150-pound senior (68 kg) need approximately 68 to 82 grams of protein per day to maintain muscular health.

- Protein-Rich Foods: Lean meats (chicken, turkey, lean beef) - Fish (salmon, tuna, sardines) - Eggs - Greek yogurt and cottage cheese - Legumes (beans, lentils) - Tofu and tempeh - Nuts and seeds

Hydration Tip For Seniors

Staying hydrated is just as important as consuming the right foods, especially during strength training and physical exercise. Dehydration can hinder your strength, endurance, and recovery, so drink plenty of water throughout the day.

Staying hydrated throughout exercise helps regulate body temperature and prevent overheating.

- Increases Muscle Function: Dehydration can cause muscle cramps and weakness. Proper hydration improves muscular function during workouts.
- Boosts Recovery: Water is essential for carrying nutrients to muscles and eliminating toxins from the body, resulting in speedier recovery.

Hydration Guidelines For Seniors Drink at least 8 cups (64 ounces) of water daily, and increase intake during exercise or hot weather.

- Before exercise:Drink 4-5ounces of water 20-30 minutes before you begin.
- During exercise: Drink 3-5ounces of water every 15-20 minutes, particularly if you're doing moderate to strenuous activity.
- After exercise: Drink 4-8 ounces of water within an hour after exercising to rehydrate and aid with recovery.

Hydrating Foods
Include water-rich items in your diet, such as cucumbers, watermelon, oranges, strawberries, and celery, as well as broths and soups, and smoothies with hydrating fruits.

Simple, Nutritious Meals To Help You Reach Your Fitness Goals
Meal planning does not have to be difficult, but it does necessitate some consideration to ensure you are obtaining the proper nutrients

to support your strength training regimen. Here are some simple and nutritious meal options to help you fuel your body for exercise, recover faster, and enjoy long-term health benefits.

- Breakfast:Greek Yogurt Parfait: Combine Greek yogurt, berries, chia seeds, and granola for a balanced breakfast high in protein, healthy fats, and fiber.

Veggie Omelet with Whole-Grain Toast:An omelette with eggs, spinach, mushrooms, and bell peppers. Combine with whole-grain bread for more complex carbs and fiber.

- Oatmeal with almond butter and banana: Oats provide slow-digesting carbohydrates, while almond butter contains protein and healthful fats.

For lunch, choose the Grilled Chicken Salad, which has mixed greens, grilled chicken, avocado, cucumbers, tomatoes, and a light olive oil dressing. Add some quinoa or chickpeas for extra protein and fiber.

- Lentil Soup and Whole-Grain Crackers:Lentils are a great source of plant-based protein and fiber, which help with muscle growth and digestion.
- The Tuna Salad Wrap:Combine tuna, Greek yogurt, mustard, and chopped vegetables. Wrap in a whole-grain tortilla for a simple, protein-rich supper.

Dinner is baked salmon with sweet potatoes and asparagus. Salmon is high in omega-3 fatty acids, which promote joint health and prevent inflammation, whereas sweet potatoes have complex carbohydrates that offer energy.

- Stir-Fried Tofu and Veggies with Brown Rice:A simple stir-fry of tofu, broccoli, carrots, and bell peppers served with brown rice to boost fiber and antioxidants.

- Turkey Chili: Lean ground turkey, kidney beans, tomatoes, and spices combine to create a robust and full meal that promotes muscle regeneration.

Snacks

- Hard-Boiled Eggs:Protein-rich and easy to prepare ahead of time.
- Mixed Nuts And Seeds: One handful of nuts contains healthy fats, protein, and energy.
- The Protein Smoothie:Combine a scoop of protein powder, spinach, almond milk, and frozen fruit for a tasty and nutritious snack.

Proper diet is essential for maximizing your strength training outcomes and ensuring your body heals completely. By focusing on a balanced diet with appropriate protein, staying hydrated, and eating entire, nutritious meals, you give yourself the best chance of success in your fitness journey. Consistency in both exercise and nutrition is critical for long-term health, vigor, and independence.

CHAPTER 10

IMPORTANCE OF REST AND RECOVERY

Rest and recovery are critical components of any exercise plan, particularly as we age. Muscles do not have enough time to renew and heal themselves without appropriate rest, which can result in fatigue, injury, and stagnation. Taking the time to relax properly helps your muscles develop stronger, keeps your mind fresh, and allows you to continue training efficiently.

Rest and recovery are crucial for muscle repair and growth. Strength training generates microscopic breaks in muscle fibers, which require rest to mend and rebuild stronger.

- Prevents Overtraining and Injury: Without adequate rest, muscles might get weary and more susceptible to injury, limiting the effectiveness of your workouts.

- Restores Energy Levels: Strength training depletes your body's glycogen stores, and rest replenishes these energy sources, allowing you to perform at your peak in subsequent exercises.
- Mental Rejuvenation: Recovery days provide a mental break, which helps to prevent burnout and maintain motivation levels.

Rest And Recovery Tips For Seniors
Schedule Regular Rest Days
Allow for 1-2 days of rest each week or engage in active recovery activities like walking or stretching to keep the body moving without overloading it.

- Sleep is essential: Make sleep a priority. Aim for 7-9 hours of quality sleep per night to help your muscles repair and your mind recharge.
- Active recovery: On rest days, do light exercises like yoga, swimming,

or walking to keep blood flowing and alleviate muscle stiffness without putting too much strain on the body.

- Hydrate and Refuel: Proper diet and hydration are critical to recovery. Make sure you're getting enough protein, healthy fats, and carbohydrates to aid with muscle regeneration.

Healthy aging entails choosing a lifestyle that benefits your health, mind, and soul. You can prepare yourself for a life of vitality, confidence, and joy by including flexibility and stretching exercises, improving your mental health through strength training, and emphasizing rest and recovery.

CONCLUSION

Strength training is not just a series of exercises; it's a gateway to a healthier, more vibrant life, regardless of age. By embracing the techniques and routines outlined in this book, you've taken a significant step toward improving your physical strength, enhancing your mobility, and boosting your overall confidence.

This journey is about more than fitness,it's about reclaiming your independence, preventing injuries, and empowering yourself to enjoy life to its fullest. With consistency, patience, and a positive mindset, the benefits of strength training will extend beyond your body, enriching your mental and emotional well-being as well.

Remember, it's never too late to start. Each small step forward is progress worth celebrating, and your commitment to health is a testament to your resilience and determination. Let this book be your guide, inspiring you to continue striving for a stronger, healthier, and more fulfilling life.

Share your journey with loved ones, inspire others to join you, and carry the message that strength training is truly transformative at any age. You are living proof that the golden years can be your strongest years.

Now, take what you've learned and make every movement a celebration of vitality, every session a step toward your best self, and every day an opportunity to thrive. Let this be the start of your most empowered chapter yet.
Your strength is your legacy.

VIDEOS

https://hasfit.com/workouts/home/senior/30-min-strength-training-for-seniors-exercise

https://go.usa.gov/xtqAy

https://youtu.be/x6wiDew4sYU?si=_neZ4q CrvoDvK4uA

https://youtu.be/Cl7E5GoFv6k?si=M56N42 Cqt6oIi0NG

https://youtu.be/9Yvl5XxvCCw?si=-hMyL Wf4YJM3Xnjx

https://youtu.be/J0vhOvj5Kms?si=wnci5v9 WDeYF-iov

https://youtu.be/QOIhn8Hjb1Y?si=NtM7Z8 Q3QNWVJncU

https://youtu.be/jlN217tjnxM?si=aGDWOp9 kOMkzsDT-

https://youtu.be/jReivdS83Mo?si=pT3JLD9
0BduD9mNY

https://youtu.be/WY0WYyxP7d0?si=0rzGD
_hiUvxm2iYp

https://youtu.be/5_xnJL5CYOQ?si=-FVeuiC
6HQsS2vVo

https://youtu.be/8CE4ijWlQ18?si=NtZHo3y
TocLJk3vH

https://youtu.be/0r6w8K6ckQk?si=Um0krup
-eh9UPdFv

https://youtu.be/5NlDKkrMn5U?si=6aS_JX
Jd4ibywouH

https://youtu.be/IdcKe52onKU?si=aKq75Fu
AN3ekVPmL

https://youtube.com/shorts/vH74Wolc0YU?s
i=JtathiU1HTdaxClL

https://youtu.be/Ev6yE55kYGw?si=INwx5wCRgWVT8vQM

https://youtu.be/pUYxcRvdal8?si=0yVUv066o6mEubT9

https://youtu.be/3RTaz95dKBo?si=wc2nIcJcjD5q55Vb

https://youtu.be/A2jUBUdbJQo?si=kMyY4C2KX82IPogr